I'm Still Here

Living Long and Loving Life
at Age Ninety Plus

David Lemon, MD

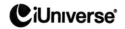

I'M STILL HERE
LIVING LONG AND LOVING LIFE AT AGE NINETY PLUS

iUniverse books may be ordered through booksellers or by contacting:

iUniverse
1663 Liberty Drive
Bloomington, IN 47403
www.iuniverse.com
1-800-Authors (1-800-288-4677)

Because of the dynamic nature of the Internet, any web addresses or links contained in this book may have changed since publication and may no longer be valid. The views expressed in this work are solely those of the author and do not necessarily reflect the views of the publisher, and the publisher hereby disclaims any responsibility for them.

Any people depicted in stock imagery provided by Thinkstock are models, and such images are being used for illustrative purposes only. Certain stock imagery © Thinkstock.

ISBN: 978-1-4917-8448-8 (sc)
ISBN: 978-1-4917-8449-5 (e)

Library of Congress Control Number: 2015920293

Print information available on the last page.

iUniverse rev. date: 12/04/2015

Contents

Acknowledgements

I'd like to thank my wife Suzanne for her help in editing this book.

I'd like to thank my father-in-law, Milo who shared his life story as an example of people living successfully to age 90 and beyond.

I'd like to especially thank my patients who've allowed me to care for them and for sharing their life stories with me.

Introduction

My name is David. I am a cardiologist. For the uninitiated, that means I am a doctor who specializes in taking care of the heart. I have been doing this for nearly forty years, so I think I know how to do my job well. I know what works and what doesn't work. I've noticed over the years that I spend more time with patients discussing "matters of the heart" more than what is "wrong with my heart". I've also noticed that I am getting older and my patients are getting older. I find them saying to me several times a day, "How long are you going to work, Doc?" or "You're not going to run out on me, are you!" I tell them, "No," and assure them that I'll be there as long as my mind works, my body doesn't give out, and my partners will put up with me. Most of them smile and seem relieved. Then we talk about their grandkids, great-grandkids, and then, if we have time, we talk about their hearts. Some leave in wheelchairs or walkers, but I hope most of them leave with a smile.

When I started my great adventure dealing with peoples' hearts, we felt that anyone over the age of seventy was "over the hill" and we would say or think the phrase, "let nature take its course." Let's just don't hurt them. Then a funny thing happened. We found out that seventy wasn't so old. We did all sorts of things to people like heart surgery and balloons and stents and they just kept coming back for more. Then we found that even eighty-year-old patients tolerated all sorts of aggressive things, and yes, they smiled through all of it. I started noticing that their clinical records indicated that numerous interventions over the years were done. They just kept moving on, thriving, adapting, and their charts got thicker and thicker. They started looking not so old as I aged along with them.

I began looking at the ages of the patients I was seeing. I realized that lately, 80 percent of my patients were Medicare age, or at least 65 years old. Then I saw that 70 percent were greater than 70 years old, a third greater than 80 years old, and yes, one or two patients were at least 90 years old. Yes, indeed, times were a changin'. This gave me an idea. Why not look at these folks greater than 90 years and see what made them tick. I had all their records. I knew their lives, their spouses, their dreams, their failings, in short, their lives. I then set about in a very deliberate way asking leading questions and trying to draw out their secrets for longevity and happiness. For more than four years I did this and recorded their responses. Over that time I accumulated responses from more than 120 folks. I would like to share with you now what I learned and how we can learn from them. Some is flattery, some is sad, some is inspiring. All of it is true. Here is their story. It all begins with my father-in-law, "Grandpa".

Chapter 1

Grandpa

My story begins and will end with "Grandpa". He is also known by those who know and love him as Milo, Mike, Pop or Dad but I will stick with how I know him, "Grandpa". He is one of those guys Tom Brokaw called part of "the Greatest Generation". Indeed he is. He has exposed and lived those values of faith, family, and friendship every day and still does to this very day. He is a child of the Great Depression. He performed physical labor much of his adult life. If something broke, he fixed it. All of his family helped fix it. He only once bought a new car; he saved his money, paid his bills and prayed to the Lord every day. He put five children through college. One of his later hobbies was to scour garage sales for tools and streets for what some people called "trash". He took some of this treasure home and usually could make that "trash" work just fine. To this day, he wants to pay his own way, help out, and contribute. He is fiercely devoted to his family. But I'm getting ahead of myself. Let's learn a little about him.

Grandpa is ninety-four. He was born in 1920 in northwest Iowa where he learned to speak only Dutch. In 1923 his family moved to Chicago and settled in a Dutch neighborhood. Several years later they moved to Cicero where he attended Timothy Christian School. After graduating from high school he began working his entire 40-year career at Illinois Bell Telephone Company. In 1943 he joined the army and spent 18 months in Algeria as a corporal. He was in the signal corps and installed communication services ahead of the advancing forces. He once had the distinction of meeting Gen. Dwight D. Eisenhower and remembers "Ike" admonishing him for improperly wearing a hat while in uniform. In 1944 he was stationed in Naples, Italy as a staff sergeant for two years. In 1951 he married the love of his life, Geraldine, lovingly called to this day, "Livey". After working in construction and splicing cable, working in manholes and climbing poles for years, he was moved indoors to the accounting office at Illinois Bell. His comments about that time were summarized, "I didn't like supervising women." Livey gave birth to the first of their five children, Suzanne, my wife and love of my life. The family moved from Chicago to suburban Westchester. As the family grew they moved to a larger house in La Grange where Grandpa lived until July 2014. In 1988 I had the good fortune to crash the party and join the group. As we speak, Grandpa has 13 grandchildren who all reflect his values and about whom he is kept updated on their lives and plans. Let's take a look at Grandpa's recent life and see if you can see yourself or your mother or dad.

Four years ago Grandpa stated emphatically, "I don't want to make any changes. I'm satisfied with my life." He recalled an incident going to church. He'd gotten out of his car but it was icy. He couldn't go forward or backward. "So I just sat down on my butt." A woman was nearby but, "She couldn't help me; she was worthless. So I rolled over and got up on my knees and finally pulled myself up." (During this period Grandpa was living alone. His wife had died several years before). He remained engaged in life. He attended Bible study regularly, made and delivered sandwiches with church members to the needy on the south side of Chicago. When his older friend, Bill could no longer drive, Grandpa drove Bill and himself to sandwich duty—he was much younger then—only in his 80's. He continued to swelter in his home in the summer refusing to turn on the window air conditioner. Many days he would make a "to-do" list. He balanced his checkbook to the penny each month. Then, as now he was oblivious to pain and yes, he would occasionally take a "header" but get on his feet and heal up again. He continued to make many of his own meals even at age 90. At that time he could remember most of the important family birthdays, knew all his neighbors and never missed church. He wanted to stay in his home and felt that going to assisted living "would be like giving up." He still did his own laundry and hung his clothing and towels on the line to dry after the dryer broke and he refused to buy a new one.

But all things can't last forever and alas, age started its relentless march. Two years ago Grandpa recounted a happening that reflects age and determination. "I was trying to get up. The chair went one way and I went the other, so I hit the floor and just laid there. Then I rolled over and after a while I pulled myself up with another chair. After all, I wanted to go for a bike ride." As Grandpa reflected on younger workers changing jobs, he said, "It wasn't that way when I worked. I could never think about leaving my job."

Two years ago we noted that Grandpa didn't seem to be doing quite as well. He was sleeping a lot. He seemed to be having increasing difficulty swallowing. Being "the doctor" and my wife being "the nurse", we wanted to know why, and boy did we undertake a journey. Various tests showed that Grandpa's esophagus was very dilated and didn't work right so the food couldn't get easily to his stomach, but instead just sat there. Sometimes it would go down, but sometimes it would come back up. One test lead to another and alas, we found he had cancer in his stomach. Thankfully, due to the skill of his GI doctors, the cancer was completely removed with a less aggressive procedure that cured the problem. The Lord was with Grandpa and his doctor that day. He still has trouble swallowing, but we are thankful he is alive to even have that problem.

Grandpa lives with us all the time now. His house in La Grange sold to the first bidder at the "asked for" price. His kids worked to get it spic and span. He says he feels like our home is now his home.

Not too long ago Grandpa decided he was going to replace the broken drain cover in our garage with my wife's assistance. He was sitting on his bike (a three-wheel trike really) and whacking away at the drain cover. Then he slid off the bike onto the garage floor. He couldn't get up. My wife couldn't get him up. She finally scooted him to the stairs and managed after several attempts to finally get him up. He then finished the job and slept the rest of the day.

Oh yes! Grandpa and his bike. It is a beautiful blue three-wheel recumbent bike. It really is magnificent. It has been a huge part of his life the past eight years. Rain or shine, winter, snow, frigid temps, nothing can keep him off the bike. It has a nice orange flag on back. Two or three times a day, out he goes. He often meets neighbors or kids on his ride. He loves children, especially babies. He lights up when he sees them. The rides have gotten shorter, but the effort is still there. Thank you, Lord, for his bike. Sometimes he has trouble getting up the incline to our driveway, but so what, a neighbor will give him a push. Some time ago he was riding in a nearby parking lot and turned too fast. Yes, you guessed it; over he went, trapped under the bike. Once again the Lord was watching over him. A nearby Good Samaritan helped him up. Yes, he got a bruised head and a bruised ego, but he lived to ride again. Later, if he hadn't returned in a few minutes from his ride my wife would go out to find him. Nowadays, she accompanies Grandpa on her bike. Should we not let him ride his bike? I think not. It is more than a bike. It gives meaning and independence to his life. May the good Lord continue to protect him.

Grandpa's days are fairly predictable now. He sleeps 10-12 hours at night and gets up about 8 am or so. He manages to get himself out of bed and with the use of a walker he inches his way to the kitchen. He will have two naps most days each 1-2 hours long. My wife as I mentioned is a nurse, and a great one. We feel he is getting "skilled care" in all respects. Grandpa has diabetes that is managed skillfully by my wife with a little input from me. We have him on the "ice cream, mashed potato, chocolate, and sausage diet." No kidding. We figure when you are 94 you should eat what you like and yes, his blood pressure and diabetes are doing just fine, thank you. He still eats too fast sometimes, leading us often to pray this is not his last meal. He has trouble getting out of a chair without help, but thanks to my lovely wife, he has help. He Skype's with his children and grandchildren several times a week and is always interested in what's going on in the family.

Grandpa loves TV and is a real channel surfer. Don't get too interested in a program because it might be gone in a moment. Who needs to speak Spanish to watch the Spanish channel?

He loves crossword puzzles. My wife spends hours helping him fill them out. That is love and devotion on her part. He recently wrote a note to one of his buddies and started it out, "I and Sue are ok."

Last week he complained that his foot was hurting him. My wife explored the situation. Wouldn't you know, he had a sock wadded up in the toe of his shoe. Ouch! That would hurt.

Often when we go out to eat or get a pizza, Grandpa insists on paying. We graciously accept, but I think he has already paid his dues.

He avidly reads his Bible. Its teachings have guided his life. He reads the Des Moines Register and Wall Street Journal cover to cover each day and is very aware of current events.

But a few things have been troubling in regard to his health. In the past he has had trouble finding the right word to say or had garbled speech. So far it is transient. We had him see a neurologist and do some tests. Apparently there is nothing to do except what we are doing now and pray that the Lord will handle it the way He sees fit. In the meantime he continues to love life. He tells us he is "living on borrowed time". Maybe so. We hope he can borrow just a little more time.

We'll return to Grandpa's saga later. Let's talk about getting "really old" and what it means to us as a nation, to families, and to the "oldsters".

Chapter 2

What are the Real Issues?

Getting old and being old depends upon who is talking and about whom you are describing. I used to think seventy was old. Now, as I approach seventy myself, I think that being old is always something in the future. In my medical practice of cardiology almost everyone is "old". My focus here is on folks over ninety years; a definition even the most forgiving person would say is "really old". Several issues are common to these "oldsters" that involve families, friends, spouses, and our nation as a whole. Let's talk frankly about some of these issues and later discuss approaches to deal with them.

I frequently have patients tell me, "Sometimes I think I have just lived too long," or "I'm living on borrowed time." When I ask them what they mean, they will say, "life is so hard". My comeback line is usually, "Yeah, but you have to be tough to be old." They will smile, but then look down at the floor and become very quiet. Then they explain, "My wife died six years ago and it's just not the same. I used to cook her oatmeal for breakfast; now I eat my oatmeal alone. I used to play golf and go to the club, but Joe and Harry and Bill are gone and wouldn't you know, they closed the damn club down. My kids come over every day and check on me. I tell them I'm fine. They even said I should move in with them. How could I do that? Last month they took my car keys away; said they were doing it for my own good. My son said that if I wanted to kill myself driving my car, ok, but he doesn't want me killing somebody else. I suppose he's right. But just between you and me, I have an extra set of keys and I'm fixing to take a little trip to the grocery store tomorrow. I'm just so tired all the time. Seems like I try to do something and I have to take a two hour nap. It didn't used to be that way. I want to be useful. I don't want to be a burden. I've always paid my own way and now, you know, I'm not worth nothing. I have trouble getting out of this "baby" chair they've gotten me and sometimes I do fall down. So far I haven't conked my head. So far I've gotten up each time, but boy, it's hard. Then there is my walker. At first I thought it was for cripples only; now I love it. It has a nice seat on it; I can just sit down anytime I want, read the paper and then get on my merry way. I like to read the paper. It makes me feel like I'm connected to the real world. Trouble is two hours later I can't remember what I read. I used to know all my grandkids' birthdays, but now I can't. I love when my grandkids come over. I like their friends. They seem so nice. I sure wish I could go back and be like them. I can't hear so well, but if you look at me and talk loud, I can make it out; and if I give them a smile they will at least think I heard them. I sometimes have trouble getting to the bathroom in time. I think I'm feeling better about myself recently. I think I am starting to adapt to this getting old thing. I don't like it, but I can't change it. I have a great family; some old guys aren't so lucky. I think God is looking out for me. He will tell me when it's time to go home. He has a place all set for me. I guess it's not time yet. If I can't drive I still like to ride along. I sit in the car, watch the people go by and look at the beautiful trees and sky. I guess I'll stick around for a while longer, the good Lord willing."

Of course, families will look at their moms and dads and their problems from a different vantage point. Maybe the narrative and issues would play out something like this. "Dad just doesn't like getting old. Maybe he should go to assisted living. I think he should move in with us, but he'll have nothing of it. He says he would be too much trouble. On one level he's right; but I owe him so much—now it's my turn. I'm afraid he will fall and hurt himself. What if he can't get up? What if he hurts himself? I could never live that down. We have him now wearing a warning device that he can push at any time and let us know if he needs help. Sometimes he forgets to put it on. I try to check on him at least twice each day. He comes over most days to eat supper or I'll bring food over to him. The neighbors are good; they check on him every day too. He can't hear the telephone anymore, so I just need to go over and check on him. My son mows his yard and my dad makes sure each time that he pays my son and makes a production of it. We have trouble convincing Dad that we want to help, that he is not a "burden", and we enjoy his company. We read the Bible together. He still likes to tell me stories of when he was young. Sometimes I'll hear the same story twice in the same day. The walker is a godsend. We take it everywhere. But then there are the days I wonder how long this will go on. He is never going to be able to hear any better or walk any better or remember things any better. He will fall I will have to get him up. Should I feel guilty about these things? Is it bad to want some free time for myself and the rest of the family? Can I safely go to the mall? Would it be bad if someday he died quietly in his sleep? I hear him calling now, no time to waste."

And then there is the doctor; that's me, or do they call us "health care providers" now? I have the luxury of seeing the oldsters, dealing with their problems and family issues, but then walking away. I can see their issues in a bit of a different light. When I went to medical school, now it seems like the dark ages, the first thing they taught us was "do no harm". In plain English that means don't make people worse trying to make them better. Every day that is an issue. Today we have what are called "appropriate use guidelines". They are intended to guide us in the decision making process. Sometimes, however, the procedure or device allowed is appropriate on paper, but inappropriate in real life situations. Sometimes life prolonging devices like cardiac defibrillators are placed in 85-90 year old people who "fit the numbers"; but common sense would say, "No way!!" Where do we stop? When is enough enough? But we cannot make a pronouncement on another person's quality of life. Our job is to let people tell us what their quality of life is and what they value. It's amazing how much you can learn if you just shut up and listen. Then there is the cost of care. Everyone knows medical care costs too much, but at the same time we want our family and loved ones to get the best. It's ok to be conservative and prudent with everyone else, "but when it comes to 'my dad', don't you dare withhold therapy unless I say so".

And so it goes. Let's turn our attention to some real people with real stories to tell. These are people who are all 90 years or older whose lives I have had the privilege to follow for the last few years.

Chapter 3

Our Typical Iowa Female Patient

Let's start with the ladies. It's Monday morning and my first patient is a woman, age 90. We will call her Mabel. What follows is a typical scenario for an interaction with Mabel.

First of all, Mabel probably lives in a small town in rural Iowa. She had been married for 60 years, but her husband died three years ago. She now lives with her married daughter who accompanies her. They both had to get up at 5 am to get ready, do the chores, and go over directions on how to get to the office. She always arrives on time, and I am always late. She has taken time to put on a nice dress, put her hair up in a bun and put on just a touch of makeup. She has her list of medicines tucked away in her purse. She is asked to fill out information on an electronic check-in kiosk, which is mind boggling even to a Rhodes Scholar. This takes at least twenty minutes on a good day. The chances are about one-in-four she will be using a walker. She hates the darn thing. Finally she gets to the examining room. Once again our nurse interrogates her at length and they chat about the grandkids, the weather, and how Mabel is feeling and doing. Mabel's daughter is hovering nearby, pen in hand and an open notebook, writing down everything the nurse says. Mabel tells the nurse that she just can't work hard anymore; she just tuckers out, and some days, "I just wish the good Lord would call me home." Her daughter interrupts saying, "Mom, you don't mean that! What would we do without you? Don't talk such nonsense." This dialogue continues for a moment until the nurse cuts the tension with, "The doctor will be in shortly." "Shortly" in medical terms could be five minutes or it could be twenty minutes.

After what seems like an eternity, I step into the room. Before I can reach out to shake her hand, Mabel chirps, "How you doing, doc?" My response is always, "Mabel, I'm supposed to ask you how you are doing." No matter how sick she is Mabel is always cheerful and conversational. This may be the only outside interaction she has had in a month. Mabel herself is always tidy, polite, sitting with her hands folded in her lap. Mabel could be 130 pounds and petite, but in Iowa she would more likely be 180 pounds and "robust". Her daughter has her notebook out with pen in hand and is just a little reserved. She doesn't quite know what to make of this. After a minute or two, we talk about Mabel's health. She constantly changes the subject and wants to talk about my health and how I'm doing. She wants to make sure I'm not going to retire and that they are not working me too hard. Her daughter interrupts, "Mom, tell him about the dizzy spells." "They are nothing," she retorts. "You worry too much. What can you expect with a 90 year old gal not worth my weight in peanuts anymore." "Now Mom, that's not true! We couldn't manage without you." This back and forth goes on for a minute. I just watch and listen for cues as to what the real issues are in her case.

Eventually we figure out that maybe Mabel's heart rhythm is going crazy; we need to have her wear a monitor to look at what might be causing this. Mabel reluctantly agrees to wear the contraption. She is skeptical we will find anything worthwhile. We do the physical exam, review her medicines, and I write down on a piece of paper exactly what we talked about and the planned workup. I give the paper to her daughter. She smiles for the first time and thanks me. With her daughter's help, we jointly wrench Mabel off the table, slide her walker in front of her, and gently head her toward the checkout station. She promptly turns the wrong way, then stops, looks at the sign, and wheels around, heading for the checkout. This total interaction has lasted about twenty minutes, so as usual I'm late for the next patient. Most of the interaction has been spent on life issues, not physical heart issues. I've learned over the years that is what is most important.

Mabel is fortunate. She has family. In Iowa, this is the norm—not in other parts of the country. She is part of family community. She has meaning to her life. She contributes. That is the key. The medicines she takes are a necessary nuisance. Mabel will continue to do well unless she falls or gets a bad case of the flu, or gets her medicines mixed up. She still wants to drive her car, fix breakfast, make the bed, and make sure no mud gets on the carpet. I told Mabel she was doing "great". She is doing great. I hope the monitor doesn't show anything bad. Oh well, on to the next patient.

Chapter 4

The Ladies

First up is Lois. What an amazing lady. She had a heart valve operation seventeen years ago and still loves life. She is 92 years old and proud of it. Lois is a hospice minister. She works full time. She refuses to slow down. She doesn't believe in flu shots. She tells me she wants "to wear our, not rust out." Two years ago she performed seven wedding ceremonies over the Christmas holiday and loved it. "I don't want to die with my boots off." She chirps when I tell her she had a pig heart valve. She retorts, "I must have had a good pig." She lives alone. She carries wood, mows two acres, and still shovels snow. She has no vision in her right eye, but still continues to drive. She says she frequently gets up at 2:30 am to minister to hospice families if necessary. She works part-time as a Walmart greeter. Once per month members of her community get together at the Firestone store and Lois cooks noodles for fifty people. Last year Lois cooked Thanksgiving dinner for twenty-nine people and for twenty-five people on Christmas Day. She tells me, "I love everything I do." Last year Lois had a bleeding problem. On the way to the emergency room she noticed she had forgotten her false teeth and made her daughter go back home and get them. She told the ER doctor they had to get her fixed up in a hurry because she had a wedding to perform the next day. Yes—she got to the wedding. To start the year 2013, Lois penned a poem for me.

From God's rich blessings we may glean.
In the year twenty thirteen.

At her last visit, Lois proclaimed, "I don't wa
They'll get you whenever you go there."

AMAZING!

This year Lois shows no signs of slowing down. She recently finished constructing a shed, canned fifty-five jars of tomatoes and had two marriage ceremonies coming up in the next week. During her lifetime, Lois took care of thirty-two foster children, adopted four children, and had one of her own. At her last clinic visit she gave me a pen. On the barrel of the pen was written, "The year 2014 is here. We will honor and praise God this year." Wow. What an amazing woman.

Ruth is a story of courage. She has severe arthritis and needs to use a wheelchair. Name a medical problem and Ruth has had it or has it now. Here is a short list: coronary bypass surgery, kidney disease, diabetes, Parkinson's disease, two knee replacements and oh yes, she has a pacemaker. That's enough to make anyone sad or discouraged. How does she do it? She tells me, "I'm glad to be alive. I always told my kids, 'If you want to work, you can find a job.'" She grew up with the Great Depression mentality. She picked cotton as a young woman, then worked for the telephone company, raised five kids, adopted one. One of her sons is a minister. She tells me all about her eleven grandkids and ten great-grandkids. Never complains. Always smiles. Tough! Tough! When I grow up that's how I want to be!

Then there is Bonnie. She is now 97 years young. She gets out every day. She is the assigned book reader for her ladies' group. She is taking a printing class at our local university. She reminds me she is a Democrat and "proud of it". She is too busy to nap. Instead, she does chair yoga and likes to give talks to her friends. She tells emphatically, "I only want to be told I'm doing well if I'm really doing well." She is doing well. She is much too busy to slow down.

Evelyn is lovely. She epitomizes a tough optimistic spirit. She doesn't like people to help her if she can do something herself. The key she says is "to work all the time and love it." She gets up every morning at 6 am. She makes 100 quilts per year and gives them to kids with cancer. She wants to stay in her home at all cost and to help people. She still shovels snow, mows a huge yard, and bakes all the time she is not quilting. Oh, in her "spare time" she does Bible studies for the prison ministry nine times per month. By the way, she is 95. I'm tired just thinking about all her energy.

Edna is a real survivor. Each time I see her she quips, "I remember you—you put a stent in my heart. I thank the good Lord every day for my stent." She still lives alone, but her kids and grandkids are over all the time. She likes to roam around Walmart and her family says they can never find her. She works in the yard using her cane to help her do the job. She reminds me that her dad lived to 103. She makes me feel good when she says with all sincerity, "You look like a kid to me." I remind her that I have seven grandkids of my own.

Anna is one tough lady. She owns a laundry, lives alone, buys her own groceries and mows her yard. She says she has fallen fourteen times in the last year. She refuses to go to a nursing home. She quips, "I can't see, I can't hear, I can't walk, but I'm ok. I always pay my help," she emphasizes. Four years ago her daughter's house burned down, so she and her six kids moved in with Anna. She tells me when it is her time she wants to die quickly without a big fuss. She is 97 years old.

Maxine is the type of person we would all like to emulate. She taught school for 43 consecutive years, mostly in a one-room schoolhouse. She still drives thirty miles per day. She has several advanced academic degrees and tells me she has visited all fifty states.

She recently visited Ireland and Italy. She likes keeping up with all the students she mentored through the years and is interested in their families and activities. She enjoys life she says. She loved being a teacher and wants to do more, but she just gets worn out. She sums up life by telling me, "I would do it all over again!" She was only 94 at her last visit.

Norma is one of the most extraordinary ladies I have had the privilege to know. She is a very young 90. She is a beautiful woman—tall, thin, and tough as nails. She recently moved off the farm, but only reluctantly. She tells me she misses feeding the cows. She played a video the days she was moving—"The Good, The Bad and The Ugly." She is a very conservative Republican. Attitude is the key she tells me. She looks at me and says, "Don't retire, just change your occupation." She still "cash rents" her farm. "Nobody in Washington knows what they're doing," she says. She loves to look up things in the encyclopedia and surprise her family with what she knows. She admits she is still "hyper" and wants to keep busy. She loves watching sports and loves former Indiana basketball coach Bob Knight. She is slowing down a little and doesn't like it a bit. If she walks up a hill and just can't continue, she sits down and puts on her oxygen and then continues. Last Spring her bridge washed out and she was stranded for a few days. No problem though; she tells me she had more time to get "all my book work done." Wow! Nothing can stop this amazing woman!

Virginia is an example of thankfulness. She emphasizes what she can do, not what she can't do. She tells me, "Each morning when I wake up I thank the good Lord for giving me one more day." She can only walk about 50 yards at a time and has to stop three times to catch her breath—but "so what" she says. "I can't pull stumps anymore, but I can garden, sew, read, and bake a mean apple pie." I think she is an inspiration to us all. She is a gutsy, thankful, young 92-year-old icon as far as I am concerned.

Hazel's story is one of "true" love. She is 92. Her husband has Alzheimer's disease. She changes his diaper three times per day and gives him his insulin two to three times per day. She feeds him, bathes him and makes sure the rails are up on his bed at night. She does this all without outside help. She always has a smile, a kind word, and is bright and cheery. On her last visit she wore a beautiful red blouse. What a wonderful lady.

Maxine is a feisty woman with a great smile. She is a "fancy lady". She doesn't like to follow advice. Up until age 93 she played golf. She wears a lot of gold rings and each has a story. She doesn't like the food at the nursing home where she lives. At age 95 she told me, "I'm ready to go any time the good Lord calls. Don't think I'm not thankful or grateful. I am blessed." But, no more driving and no more golf. "Without books I would go crazy," she says. Now at age 96, things are not going well. Her weight is down seventeen pounds. She still has a smile. At the end of our visit she tells me with a sneaky smirk, "My friend stopped eating and taking her medicines. Sounds like a good idea to me." All good things have to end sometime I guess.

Daisy is stone deaf. At her last visit she cracked me up. She told me with all sincerity, "If I make it to 95 we will go have a beer." Okay, maybe so.

Mary is 95 and just too tough to die. She falls and is confined to a nursing home, but she refuses to give in. She still drives, watches TV, and exercises thirty minutes per day. She loves college basketball. "I don't like crabby people," she says. She still gets her nails manicured and never misses an appointment. She will live until she dies.

Annette is 90. She has a lot of difficult medical problems. She told me, "I don't want to feel this way. I didn't bargain on living this long. Doctor, take care of yourself so you can take care of me." That really hits home, doesn't it.

Estella is a real ball of energy. She is 93. She is a retired schoolteacher. Her sister is 100, so she thinks she will hang around for a while. She provides dinners for her church and for funerals. She has her own greenhouse. She has hiked parts of the Appalachian Trail many times. She still walks thirty minutes per day, every day. She still lives alone on the farm since her husband died five years ago. She rode on a float in her last local Fourth of July parade. She sums her philosophy of life by telling me, "I have an honest tan; I have earned it."

Flossie is her own person and clearly is "the boss". She refuses to slow down even though she is short of breath. She refuses a blood thinner and won't use a walker. She won't let her husband do dishes or help with the housework. "I should be able to do that," she says. "I will not take a nap." But then she says, "Why am I so tired?" She is "only" 92. Oh well, you can't please them all.

Pauline just turned 100. She grew up on a farm and always took care of herself. She never drank alcohol or smoked cigarettes. "I appreciate being able to do things on my own," she says. "I'm happy with simple stuff." She still drives, listens to CD's, and loves to watch the news. "I always want to do what's right." I think one of her quips sort of sums up her ability to adapt. "They tried to get me some false teeth. They weren't right though so I decided not to eat so much meat and I'm doing ok." I think she is telling us to adapt to our circumstances, don't complain, just do it. It seems to have worked pretty well for her.

Louise is 91. To say it kindly, she is very unique. She goes to the casino once a week. "No one can deceive me," she says. "They told me when I moved into the living quarters that it was a good Christian place. I told them I've got bad news—I'm a Roman Catholic." She has a lot of unique thoughts on how to deal with life:
Dear God in heaven, help me.

Holler and scream, then work it out.

Always take three deep breaths.

No pain pills, I can take it.

She has no family around. The next quip out of her mouth, "I'm the one who takes care of 'good old dad.'" She says she's tough, and I believe it.

I saw Marian in the office last week. She brightened my day and reminded me why I love being a doctor. She is now 93 and looks and acts like she is 75. She finally retired last year as a vocational consultant. She still helps out at a local retirement facility to cheer up the "old people". She takes classes at the local university. She walks daily even though she is unsteady, and on a bad day admits she needs to use a walker. She has no intention of slowing down. She makes no excuses. She loves life. She currently is reading a book about not getting old. I believe it was called, "Live Long, Die Short".

Seeing these women as patients is very inspiring. Common themes pop up again and again. The most important ones are family and feeling useful and relevant. How are the kids doing? Are they coming over for dinner? Do you think Betsy will marry that guy? I hope she doesn't move far away. I hope everyone likes the jelly I made…and so on. Never do they acknowledge their age. Never do we joke about getting old. Never do we talk about changing any aspect of their daily routine. Being a "busybody" is a full time job. They all have their hair done and dress up to come see me. They are not angry or demanding. They are thankful. They believe in God and aren't afraid to tell me about the beliefs that guide their lives and dreams. In short, their lives often reflect the formula we should all follow to enjoy long and fruitful lives.

Chapter 5

Typical Guys Over 90

Okay. Let's look at the guys. Let's start by painting a picture of a typical 90-year-old Iowa farmer who comes to see me. First of all, he doesn't want to be here. His family "made him" come in. The fact that he made it to age 90 is in itself very unusual. Guys usually meet their Maker five to ten years earlier than the ladies. He is probably 5'8" to 6 feet tall and weighs from 210-310 pounds. He probably still has his cap on, probably in coveralls and "slightly" worn boots. His wife, who is a young 85 and their eldest daughter are sitting there dutifully; hands folded and very attentive. He asks me, "How you doing doc?" before I can speak. I tell him, "Just fine," and ask him what brings him here. "My car; what do you think?" He then winks and laughs. "This 'female doctor' said I had a bad heart and need to see a heart doctor. The wife insisted I come." The next ten minutes are spent trying to extract some hint of what is going on with him. He tells me, "I can still do what I want but they all want me to slow down." Gradually he concedes that he "might be" slowing down a bit, yeah maybe he does cough a bit, yes his boots are a little tight, but "I can still drive the tractor and sit in the combine." I ask him about any medicines he takes. He retorts, "Ask the wife, I don't keep track. They don't help anyway. Why waste good money on an old fart like me anyway?" His wife and daughter scold him as he blushes and sheepishly gives me a sly grin. He and I banter back and forth. I tell him I grew up in a small Iowa town and baled hay and "walked the beans" as a teenager. Immediately he brightens up and is more attentive. Slowly I extract the fact that he has heart failure and we come to some mutually agreeable way to proceed. Never does he let his guard down completely. Never does he concede that he is "all that sick." "No, I won't learn the names of my medicines. That's her job," he says and points to "the wife". "I never was big on medications. Just fix me up, Doc, or throw me in the trash." I know he really means it. I know he would be lost without "the wife" and "the daughter". I know that he knows he is blessed to have them around and attentive. Over the next two weeks he will have blood tests, an echocardiogram, and a treadmill test. He will be started on medications and they will be adjusted. All through the process, he will be dependent on his wife and daughter. Never will he concede that he "really needs the stuff". But he comes back! He asks me about my family and about those "dad gum politicians in Washington". Once in a while just for a few seconds, he will become quiet and pensive and look at "the wife" and smile ever so slightly. I know he truly loves this woman. Then he will slip back into his gruff role. We part with a mutual slap on the back and he says he "might" come back as he winks. He turns for the exit, usually turning in the wrong direction. "The wife" scolds him; he turns around, follows her and waves at me as he turns the corner.

Chapter 6

Some Pretty Good Guys

Let's start with Bob. Bob is now 93 and a very good 93. He is a prior Iowa AAU Age Champion at running distances up to three miles. He weighs the same as he did at age 20. He prides himself as the "oldest walker" at the local country club. He still power walks five miles a day and plays 18 holes of golf every day in the summer. He also does one hour of calisthenics every day with 100 push-ups followed by 100 sit-ups. Wow! He says he sleeps ten hours per day and feels good. Well, you say, he has no problems, but not true. He is blind in his right eye, has a pacemaker and has blockages in all three of his coronary arteries. He allows himself one alcoholic drink per day and three cups of coffee. His small wife looks as good as he does. He tells me "life is good". I tell him, "You have earned it. See you next year." Clearly the lesson here is attitude. He wills himself to do well, is consistent, optimistic, proactive. I wish I could bottle it!

James is a sweet man. He never gives up. Jim is 93. He laments he can't dance as much anymore. "I get dizzy," he says. "I just can't make it all the way around the floor." He still walks 45 minutes every day using his walker. One day he went three-fourths of a mile using his walker. He loves to walk the aisles at Walmart. He watches his weight. Jim has a great attitude. He will live until the day he dies and smile all the while.

Wayne is your typical "tough guy" who is really a warm and fuzzy pushover. He is a survivor of an incident in World War II when his parachute did not open. His back has hurt since then. No problem. He is also a survivor of colon cancer, meningitis, coronary bypass surgery, two knee surgeries, and numerous back surgeries. "So what." He still dances and plays golf. He reads large print books. He tells me, "I am blessed and I know it. I can still hold my whiskey but I can't hold my water. I'm ready to go when the good Lord calls me." He sings in the "Sun City Quartet." He loves to talk politics and religion with the boys and does crossword puzzles when he has time. He is constantly telling his family not to worry about him. Seems like he has life figured out pretty well so far. But he is still "young"—only 90.

Walter is another remarkable gentleman. At the end of World War II he and his troops were stranded eight miles behind Russian lines. He was a tank commander. Somehow they got out. He was injured three times and awarded the Silver Star. He showed me his shrapnel wound. He can still walk 1.75 miles in twenty-eight minutes. He rides his bike nine miles at a time and drinks fourteen cups of coffee a day. "After exercise I always come home with a good sweat," he says. Sixty-two years after the war has been over he still wakes up at night fighting the war. "I'm the last one left; the others are gone," he says. He has been diagnosed as having PTSD. He wears an American flag on his shirt. We are very grateful to you, Walter, and owe you and guys like you our freedom.

Maynard is a living legend and an Iowa icon. He will be 95 years old soon. He is a painter of wildlife and is world renown. He is also a humble man with more than his share of wisdom. Thirteen years ago he survived an operation on his heart. Three years ago he told me, "If I can't paint they might as well plant me. You need to have a goal you never quite achieve to keep you going." He gives his kids paintings of ducks each year and tells them that all he does is add one duck to the painting each year. I have the privilege of having one of his prints hanging in my home office. Two years ago he told me, "When I paint, things slow down and I relax." He was still golfing, hunting, and fishing. "I'm coasting down the back nine holes of life, but I get to hit twice as many shots," he says. Because of a tremor he now uses two hands to paint. No problem. He says he is doing his 35th painting for a guy he knows. "I've had a great life and have done what I want," he says. He laments the family won't let him drive all the way to Florida anymore. Last year he said he was starting to slow down. He told me, "When I get up in the morning I really want to go back to bed, but I say to myself, 'get up you lazy so and so.' I paint, and I'm fine." He told me his paintings were going to be displayed alongside Ding Darling's at Iowa State University. My wife and I went to the event to see them. At this year's appointment what do you know, he is still painting.

Hugh is 96 years old. He was a pilot in World War II. He knew my parents. His son was my classmate in high school. He admits he is getting unsteady when he walks on the treadmill. He tells me his wife told him, "You're going to fall; I can't get you up. I guess the coyotes will just eat you." Still he persists. Unfortunately he is beginning to develop heart failure. He still drives his car. He still wants to ride his tractor. He is mentally very sharp. His son Jim was with him at his last visit. We all know that without some sort of intervention on Hugh's aortic valve, he will die soon. We spend at least thirty minutes going over a new procedure that is less risky for folks in this situation. Hugh and his son are going home to think about it. It is a common scenario for me. When do we say enough is enough? I don't have the answer to that question.

Lester will soon be 96. He likes to go ballroom dancing with his 90-year-old girlfriend. He is talkative, involved, and very animated. He had a heart procedure thirteen years ago. He is the author of quite an entertaining book. He cooks and bakes his own bread. He drives his own car. "I don't eat that damn white bread," he quips. "Life has been interesting," he says. He has thirteen great-grandchildren. With the birth of each child he buys the birth weight of the child in chocolate and distributes it to the family. He has a unique take about heaven. He tells me he thinks it will be like trying to learn to read all over again. He admits his girlfriend is developing Alzheimer's disease and he is convinced it's because of the hair coloring she uses. As he left the office the other day he said in parting, "If something happens to me, that's ok, I've had a full life." Indeed you have. We all should be so blessed.

Joseph is a unique gentleman. He had a coronary bypass operation twenty-four years ago. His wife is in a nearby nursing home and he visits her every day. His hobby is picking up empty and discarded soft drink bottles. He has kept a ledger. He currently has picked up over 150,000 in his lifetime. He tells me it is 1200 steps around the block and 180 steps from his car to his wife's room. He tells me, "I'm satisfied if I die tomorrow." An interesting take on life I think.

Verle is a real jewel. He has survived three separate operations on his thoracic aorta. He once blacked out while driving his car. It was determined that his heart rate had slowed down too much because he'd gotten his medicines mixed up and had gotten toxic side effects. He and his wife have been the loves of each other's lives since the second grade. He used to raise 100 Angus cattle but can't quite do that anymore he says. He and his wife adopted twin sons when they were nine months old. One now is an investment broker. The other has her doctorate degree. He and his wife still shovel the driveway together even though he has to wear oxygen. He tells me, "I wish I could still farm full time." I tell him he is doing just fine. He will soon be 91.

Herbert is a stubborn, but likeable typical tough Iowa boy. He doesn't like medicines and takes them when he feels like it. He refused a blood thinner because his friend told him not to take it. He is upset because, "They are always changing the color of the pills." He can't see a lick and his wife has to drive him everywhere. He doesn't like his eye doctor because he told Herbert there was nothing else he could do. He says his wife has to swear at him a lot because he doesn't do what she wants him to do. He then breaks into a big grin. I know his game. He really is a big fuzzy marshmallow.

Albert is a real jokester. He is always saying things that are outrageous and quotable. He delivers the "Shopper" every morning in his small rural Iowa town and doesn't like to come to Des Moines. He has a nice laugh and is always relaxed. He mentors fifth and sixth graders at his church. He has finally consented to use a walker. My favorite quote from him is so typical: "I asked the devil if he wanted me—he said "No". I asked the Lord if He wanted me—He said, "No". That's why I'm here. Well Albert, stick around a while longer. He is only 91.

John is a very thankful man. He had a coronary bypass operation thirty-six years ago. For years he has made it a practice to visit post-operative patients to cheer them up. He has a great memory and is so thankful to be alive. He quips, "I think I've seen all you doctors over the years." At the thirty-year anniversary of his bypass surgery he personally contacted the surgeon and thanked him for saving his life. His joy and thankfulness are contagious and better than any medicines we can give him.

Hal is now 90. He is the epitome of class. Soft spoken, dressed to the hilt, informed, thin, follows suggestions, suntanned. He appears to be about 75 years old. About twenty-five years ago I did an angiogram on Hal. He had a very high risk narrowing in one of his coronary arteries. He did not want surgery. I did not want to risk putting in a stent. I said we would try medicines. Well, twenty-five years later he is doing fine. I guess it must have worked. He is a real stickler for details. He recently told me, "There are 168 hours in a week and you tell me your patients can't find four hours a week to exercise? Give me a break!" His latest project is one where he and a friend have developed a product that can be fed to cattle to decrease the amount of methane they produce and reduce global warming. I hope it works. And Hal, I hope you never change.

James lives what he professes. He sings in the church choir. The other day he saw a sad woman sitting alone in one of the pews at church. He told her to go ahead and take communion. She did. Later, after church she came out to thank him and they both cried. Recently he sold his trailer home and gave five thousand dollars from the sale to each of his children. Each Christmas he gives his kids $1000 and tells them to use it for others. He says all he wants to do is God's work. I admire this man.

Robert is a typical guy who just keeps getting by, although I'm not sure how. He gets up at 6 am every day. He still mows two acres with a push mower and walks two miles a day. He has been married for 72 years. "The wife" is the boss. He has no idea what his medicines are and even what his heart problem is, but his wife does. She tells him to slow down, so he speeds up. He still drives and she rolls her eyes when he tells me this. They are quite the pair. Lord protect this man or should I say, Lord protect his wife so she can protect him.

Harry is 94 years old. His wife has severe Alzheimer's disease and he is the sole care provider for her. She is a "24 hour a day job", he says. "I want to work but I just get pooped out. The golden years haven't been so golden lately," he laments. To pass the time he plays solitaire and watches television with the sound off because his wife cannot tolerate the sound. He loves "Wheel of Fortune" and "The Lawrence Welk Show". Recently he said something I haven't yet deciphered, "Let your guard down and you're gone." I hope he finds some peace.

Russell is 90 years old. He is sad and lonely, but covers it well with jokes. He likes Fox News. He is "interested" in religion and faith, but "wants proof". "I sure hope it's real," he says. He claims he is not quite ready to die just yet. He is always interested in my opinion. He said an interesting thing the other day. "I know you're a doctor, but are you a pastor or something like that?" I told him I wasn't but took it as a compliment. He smiled.

Robert is 92. He is wasting, can barely speak, and uses oxygen all the time. All his body systems are failing. He tells me, "I don't want to die but I'm ready to die. I have a strong faith in God. The doctors said I would be dead two years ago but here I am. I just want you to give me some hope." I'll try Robert, I'll try.

Paul is 98. He thinks he may be slowing down a bit. He has seven major cardiovascular problems but he just keeps going. He is a university professor. You guessed it—he is still working four hours a day. He tells me they still want him around. His mind is sharp. He is very witty and humorous. He loves life and wants to work until he dies. Major medical issues are just inconveniences, nothing more. I told him to keep working, don't get lazy, and oh yes, "I'll see you next year."

The stories and words from these men are refreshing and inspiring, but not always typical of a lot of very elderly men. In most cases, men do not age well. They tend to complain a lot more than women. Men are defined by their ability to do productive work, be it physical or mental. This trait does not subside much with age. Unfortunately, aging diminishes our physical and mental abilities and takes no prisoners. Most men have fewer friends than their female counterparts. Their friendships are often based on shared physical activities like golf, bowling, boating, or biking. These activities become harder and harder to maintain. This often results in a negative attitude and broken relationships. They tell me, "I shouldn't have retired," or "my son doesn't want me to help him with the crops anymore," or "I should have taken better care of myself when I was young," or "I should have taken that trip to Alaska," or "I don't want to give up; I'm just so damn tired all the time. Doc, what's wrong with me? Am I a hopeless case?"

Occasionally, bad habits from their youth can be revisited for elderly men. Alcohol abuse can be a real problem. Refusing to take prescribed medications or deliberately refusing medical advice is their way of asserting some sense of control. With time, most old guys eventually reinvest their lives and fall in line. The anger cools, life looks better, and they may even take a walk with "the wife" and their dog.

Chapter 7

Wit and Wisdom

I have noticed that my patients are always teaching me things and making me rethink a lot of my cherished "truths" and dogma. I am truly convinced that with age comes wisdom, wit, and perspective. Maybe it's simply a matter of more experience, more mistakes, more redo's and more time. In any event, with age comes freedom. At age 90 you don't have to prove anything. You've already done it and survived. Most of your friends and peers have long ago met their Maker. You know you've climbed the mountain and now you are walking down the other side. I would like to share some of these words of wisdom I have heard my 90 year-old patients share with me and try to decipher what the are saying to all of us.

William told me, "When I look in the mirror I don't see that old guy looking back at me." Well neither do I. We see what we think we are—be it young, handsome, worried or happy. I think he is telling us that the person in the mirror is truly what our mind and soul and inner being see, not just a reflection of our outer appearance. What do you see in the mirror?

Lois told me, "I want to wear out, not rust out." Irving said to me, "Live long but don't get old." Virginia proclaimed, "Getting old isn't for sissies!" I think each of these four individuals are saying pretty much the same message—be tough, resilient, take no prisoners, let me alone so I can get back to work. I love it!

Then there are the many who express thankfulness in poetic but everyday language that leaves one almost speechless.

John told me, "I can get up every morning. I have something to eat and I have a good wife. What more could you want? I will live forever. Forever is when my heart stops." Can't argue with that.

Allyn tells me, "I would do it all over again. At least I'm on the right side of the sod."

Thomas told me, "Don't get too excited about anything. Be thankful for the next day."

Virginia said, "Each morning when I wake up I thank the good Lord for giving me one more day." Yes, Virginia, my sentiment exactly.

Clyde's comments are truly words to live by. "You need to approach life with an attitude of forgiveness if you are going to be happy."

And then there are the funny comments and attempts at barroom humor that are wonderful.

Ed had this advice for me. "Get yourself in life where you don't have to wear socks anymore."

James told me with a straight face, "Better be seen than viewed." (As in the casket?)

One old farmer was tired of hearing my lecture on tobacco and he turned to me and said, "Chewing tobacco ain't so bad; I don't know anybody who died from second hand spit!" That really shut me up.

Doug told me, "Doc, if I make it to 95, we will go have a beer."

Ken told me in reference to quitting his job at age 90, "I've got the 'tire' thing down. I've got to work on the 're'."

Yvonne has never been hospitalized. When I told her that was wonderful, she retorted, "First time my mother saw a doctor she died." Gulp!

J. Paul told me, "The hardest thing I can do is nothing."

But we all know that life is no bed of roses and age does steal our energy, our friends, and family die or move away and meaning to our lives is sometimes hard to attain. Listen to these fine folks reflect on this.

Harry told me, "The golden years aren't so golden."

Annette reflected, "I don't want to feel this way. I didn't bargain on living this long. Doctor, take care of yourself so you can take care of me."

Amos told me the other day, "When it comes time that I can't take care of myself, then it's time to move on."

Anna said, "I can't see, can't hear, can't walk, but I guess that's ok."

And then there are the old-timers who like to give sage advice and tell you and me how we should live our lives. More often than not, they are right.

Frances told me last year, "We all know it—it's not hard—moderation, a good diet, and family are the keys."

Robert was very specific. He got out a piece of paper and from memory wrote down the keys to a good life.

1. Be happy
2. Go to church
3. Keep busy
4. Play games
5. Don't worry too much
6. Take fish oil
7. Have kids around
8. Have a good wife

Wow!

Wendell said one day, "Don't lie awake worrying about the stock market. If it tanks, we all tank, so go to sleep."

And then there are the heartfelt comments from patients.

Bonnie told me, "I know my day is coming, but I'm not going to sit around and wait for it."

Margaret told me, "You try for me so I try too." When I hear that, I realize that I am the one blessed and privileged indeed to try to help these folks.

I talked to a gentleman at church. When he asked, I told him I was a doctor. I asked him how old he was. He proudly told me he'd just turned 90. He seemed very introspective and then said if he had to do it all over again he would do three things differently.

1. Risk more
2. Reflect more
3. Do something that would live beyond him.

I told him he still had time. He laughed and walked away.

I'll finish this chapter with something Bob told me that I hope I will never forget. He said, "I don't want to die, but I'm ready to die. I have a strong faith in God. The doctors said I would be dead two years ago, but here I am. I just want you to give me some hope."

Chapter 8

I Still Want To....

I'd like to explore another dimension of getting really old. I have the perspective of a doctor. I've had the privilege of following some on these "old-timers" for 20-30 years as they've navigated their way through the highs and lows of dealing with life in general and heart disease in particular. During those years, they have often revealed their innermost fears, plans, obsessions, and family crises. They've also revealed to me many reflections on getting old. Comments I have heard again and again reflect common themes that deserve discussion and further explanation. I have told you about some of the amazing examples, but let's face it; most of us are pretty average. We have common issues, foibles, prejudices, and life matters. Let's explore some common themes, my patients' take on life, and my understanding of what they are telling me.

The first category of response to getting old I will call the "I don't want to" response. All of us do this every day. It is our way of stating our independence and general displeasure in our perception of how things are going and the "unfairness" of restrictions or burdens imposed on us by others. We see it in toddlers; it mellows somewhat as we age, and wouldn't you know, it comes roaring back as we get nearer the finish line. At least once a day I hear, "I don't want to take those 'blanket-blank' medicines. They cost too much. Besides, they don't work." And I respond, "How do you know they don't work if you don't take them?" "Well, I just know," he or she says. "Besides, my cousin Johnnie died after he took them." "How about trying just a couple of the medicines and see how it goes?" I respond. "Besides that I suppose you want me to know the names? That's 'the wife's' job," he retorts. "Maybe just recognize the names and carry a list," I say. And on it goes. Gradually we compromise. Yes, he agrees he will take "those cheap ones" but not the expensive ones. "The wife" will make a list and yes he will carry it in his billfold. Whew! One small limited victory for "the doctor". Eventually he will come around. We've got to go slow. Tell him you don't like taking medicines either, but what's a guy going to do if he wants to feel better?

Iowans are a tough breed. They will not voluntarily ask for help. You have to tell them that it's okay, that it helps their family to help them. If you put it in that context it goes better. But face it; if you're old and you ask for help it means you are less than whole and sliding down a slippery slope. Help means dependence on others, loss of control, and a downward spiral. My job is to convince them that asking for help gives them a chance for increased independence and a better life and more opportunities. Most people respond favorably if it is stated in positive terms, more mobility, social interaction, and overall quality of life.

One of the hardest activities to give up is driving a car. Would you like it if someone told you that you could no longer drive? Driving a car means freedom to explore, to be part of society, to be mobile, to be spontaneous, and to be in control. Taking this privilege away can be devastating. It works best if a doctor makes the suggestion and ties it to a medical illness, not just age. It doesn't work so well if the family makes a mandate. It is also important that a caregiver or family member assures the person they will consistently be there to get them to their prior commitments like going to church, having coffee with the boys, or playing bridge with the girls. It doesn't happen overnight, but with compassion and consistency, most oldsters reluctantly admit that it's a pretty good idea. A good alternative is to have the oldster accompany a family member when they run errands. They feel included in what's going on, it helps fill in downtime, and keeps them informed on family activities.

Then there is the whole list of trying to change lifelong behaviors like stopping smoking, drinking less alcohol, or backing away from the dinner table. Once again this is about loss of control. The usual response is, "Doc, it hasn't killed me yet; what else can I do? Are you going to take that away too?" No! I'm not going to take that away. Here common sense needs to prevail over "guidelines". It really is about quality of life. Personally, I hope Mr. Jones has a stiff shot of whiskey one minute before he joins the Lord forever.

Another common control issue is whether to use a walker. To most individuals it seems to be embarrassing and a stigma. Often it takes a good hard fall on the fanny or a huge black eye or knot on the head to even consider it. I think the perception is changing, though, and once an elderly person uses a walker, they won't put it away. It's all in how you market it. I tell people they get more independence and more mobility and therefore can do more for themselves without asking for help.

The last "I don't want to" is the most important. When I hear it, I feel sad. I just can't bear to hear the lament, "I don't want to be a bother or a burden." This is a state of mind that tells us, "I'm not worth the effort. I can't help out, I don't have value; why am I even here?" We all want to have value and meaning and contribute to our families and friends. It doesn't mean we load our oldsters up with anti-depressants and platitudes, it means we will help them find activities that do contribute and give meaning to their lives. We all can benefit from the wisdom and experience of older folks. If we as a society don't value this, we are in trouble.

If older folks sometimes send negative vibes with, "I don't want to," they also reflect the need to say the opposite, "I want to." Their assertions are telling you and me that they want to be in the game, part of what's going on, and don't want to be left behind or discounted. The first and most overt expression of the need is for the oldster to say, "I want to be independent." What does it mean? It can mean a lot of things. Examples are balancing the checkbook, deciding on what clothes to wear, when to shower, what to eat for breakfast, what TV station to watch. All of this may seem to be trivia if your life isn't characterized by these decisions as major events. If we take away these daily choices, we devalue the person and their ability to choose and have control. Often, the well-intentioned relative or caregiver is trying to help, but little by little, more and more self-worth is taken away. Let them eat chocolate for breakfast! Let them wear shorts in January!

One of the most important "I want to's" is the universal expression or desire of an older person to stay in their own home. It is their foundation, their memories, their place of refuge. No one wants to lose that. Every room, every picture, every trinket has a story, a tie to the past and link to the present. I have universally observed my patients take a very much more pessimistic view of the world if leaving their homes comes to pass. We as doctors and nurses and caregivers need to make the transition as painless as possible. We need to bring along the old house to the care center. This may mean pictures, furniture, trips back to the old neighborhood, old friends stopping by, or just reminiscing about good times and assuring them the "new place" will also have great stories that are just waiting to unfold. It takes time, but gradually a new mindset can be established so everybody can move on.

Another "I want to" that I hear a lot is the need to help out. "I want to pay for lunch." "Can I help you carry that in?" "Can I watch the grandkids?" Again, it is a cry out to us. "Let me be relevant!

Yes, I am old, but I can do it, just watch me." They see themselves as still 35 years old with gusto and swagger. The changes as we age are slow. We cannot even notice them until someone else points out our deficiencies and limitations. All of us have a defense mechanism. Let's don't take that away from our older folks. Emphasize how well they function, how amazed we are at their intellect, experience and good common sense and all the things they do better than we can do. Let them pay for lunch. Let them help wash the car. We will all feel better for the effort.

I find that older people universally tell me about their grandkids and their desire to see them achieve some milestone event—graduation from college, get a job, get married, have a child. I think that older people tend to relate to their grandchildren often better than their own children. I think this is in part because they are farther removed from their day-to-day care and hear only the good stuff. I think perhaps it is also a wish to be young like they are and see themselves when they were young. Besides, they don't have to change their diapers, drive them to school, and ground them when they misbehave.

The "I don't want to" and the "I still want to" attitude reflect a balance and leads to a state of mind or life outlook that can be hard to separate from the disease state. For instance, "I can't sleep" or "I'm tired all the time" can reflect anxiety or depression or a whole host of disease processes. It often leads to repetitive, expensive testing with equivocal and not useful conclusions. I've learned to respond to the quip, "I need a nap every day," with "so do I" and "that's normal", not four hundred dollars worth of testing.

When you are ninety years old you aren't supposed to be able to hear and see normally. In fact, you're not supposed to be alive. I don't even use the term "Alzheimer's disease" anymore; I prefer the term "old timers'" disease. I liken it to a car; there are lots of miles on the engine, the tires, and the frame, so this stuff needs some "body work". When I tell my patients this they seem to relax and look at their "equipment failure" in a different perspective.

I find that personality traits often become more accentuated with age. Older people may hide them better, but in the moment they come roaring back. As I told you earlier, my wife was working on a garage drain problem with my then 93 year-old father-in-law, and things weren't progressing. He was sitting on his three wheel recumbent bike directing the job. My wife asked him after a while if maybe they should try to fix it another day or get a plumber. He looked at her indignantly and snapped, "So you want to quit?" A flood of memories of her old family fix-it jobs came back. They didn't quit. They got it fixed; but she almost broke her back trying to get him on his feet again after sliding from the bike to the garage floor.

You may laugh or nod in recognition of such an example. I think it reflects what we all do. We are constantly redefining and attempting to establish who we are. We all want to "still do it". "I can still drive a tractor," "I can still make my bed, be useful, help others. Let me do it. I don't need your help." This attitude can be helpful or risky. If it leads to new interests or hobbies, then it gives older folks ways to fill in time gaps and sharpen motor skills and memory. Reading the newspaper, reading books, doing crossword puzzles, joining a church group, or simply checking up daily on kids and grandkids' activities gives meaning and purpose to life.

My father-in-law likes to ride along in the car when my wife runs errands. He will sit in the parking lot and watch people go by. If he sees small children he is delighted and will smile and wave at them. The child may be receptive or scared to death, but you get the idea.

We all have regrets. The older we get, the more time we have to ruminate over past mistakes and shortcomings. Unfortunately

or fortunately, as the case may be, they define who we are, how we approach each day, and how we see the world. Time and again I hear an oldster say, "My friends are all dead; I'm the last one left. I don't' go out for coffee anymore." There is a void that is hard to fill. "I wish I would have spent more time with the kids when they were young. They don't call much anymore." You can hear in their voice the sense of isolation and regret. I hear this especially from men. They often come in alone, or maybe a skilled care worker accompanies them. These are the folks who need our support as doctors and nurses. They don't need more tests. They need human contact and a voice of encouragement. They need us to be their friend. Another way I hear this expressed is the quip, "I didn't know I'd live this long, and if did, I would have done things a little differently." This is both humbling and sad. We as doctors often have to ask ourselves this question, "Is this me in a few years?"

Men especially do not thrive well when their wives die, unless they have family members who step in and help. In general, men are not good joiners, or conversationalists. They are "doers". Well, when you can't "do it", I guess you need to be able to talk about "When I could do it." Their lives are often divided into "what we used to do" and now "I don't do it anymore." This has to be verbalized. We as health care workers can't "fix it," but we can allow them to talk, even encourage them to express their feelings. It's often the first time that anyone has told them it's okay to remember, to have regrets, to have "should have's" and "could have's" and not feel like an ogre.

Sometimes these insecurities can lead to some negative consequences. I occasionally see and hear from family members that their parents are angry all the time. They act out in childish ways. They intentionally defy medical advice. They may curse and snap at loved ones. They may scowl and say, "Don't you tell me I can't do it," and stomp away. It really is a cry for help. "Somebody listen to me; somebody value me." Then we as doctors and family and society have to respond to them, not just in words, but also in our attitudes and actions, that they do indeed matter.

As they say, time is the best teacher—and so it is. Most ninety year-olds adapt. The proof is obvious. They have traveled down a long path to get where they are now. Somehow they have weathered the trials of illness, regrets, disappointments, and lost opportunities, but to reach age ninety, there have to be a lot of positives along the way. The positives have to outweigh the negatives. Adaptation is a process. It doesn't happen overnight. Perhaps the thinking would go like this: I can't solve corporate issues and decisions, but I can do the daily crossword puzzle in the paper. I can watch TV and be involved in politics and shout at the screen or applaud. There are a lot of good old movies and boy, those ladies still look good. I can read as much as I want and what I want. If I don't like a book, I'll just stop reading it—no pressure. I can Skype and keep up with my kids and grandkids. I can go to church. I can play bridge with the girls and maybe we can bake something and donate it to the homeless. Life is pretty good. Maybe getting old isn't so bad after all.

And so it goes. We all learn how to get old. Some actually survive getting old and live to tell us about the journey.

Chapter 9

Our Home is Your Home

Living to age ninety and beyond is hard work. It takes some help from others along the way. In some instances, it can get very lonely if family and friends and spouse are no longer available to give guidance and help with daily chores, appointments, and basic needs.

When we age, things that used to be easy no longer seem so easy. Getting out of a chair, walking, managing stairs, dressing, bathing, balancing the checkbook, remembering appointments—all are major events. None of this can be addressed in a vacuum because each family will address it differently. Past experience and memories will color how today's events unfold. As a doctor, I get daily snapshots of some of the dynamics, all be it, just snapshots. We doctors and society often refer to the relationship we see as "caregiver" and "patient". It sounds so clean and clinical. If you are a son or a daughter, you are much more than a "caregiver". If you live in an extended care or independent living environment with persons assigned to your care and responsible to assure that your needs are met, then these are caregivers. In either situation, it all boils down to relationships, daily needs, memories, hopes, fears, regrets, joys, and thankfully, "selective" memory of past events.

Family members can share the responsibility for taking care of Mom or Dad. It presents a tangible way to give back to those who influenced you as you negotiated all the ups and downs of daily life. Past birthdays, family trips, ballgames, family gatherings can be relived—"do you remember when"—can lead to a two-hour rendition of how they saw it. Time has a way of smoothing out the rough spots and putting a positive spin on touchy subjects leaving everyone feeling better. We still can use some advice from Mom or Dad, even if they are over 90.

But taking care of, or better yet, helping the very elderly is hard work. Taking a shower may become a major event. Clothing needs to be laundered, the walker needs to be nearby, the shoes need to be tied, the food has to be "just so". No, I can't go on vacation right now; Mom needs me here. Some days one can think, "Am I a prisoner in my own home? Does Mom or Dad realize how this has altered my life and the lives of all the family? Why did he say that?" And then it passes, the sun comes out, Lawrence Welk reruns come on the television, and life is good once again. Yes, a full range of emotions, some guilt, some thankfulness, all a part of helping parents negotiate their daily lives and problems.

The family of one of my patients shared the story of caring for their father. It's not pretty, but it's real and rings true to a lot of families.

John's Personality Changes:

Dementia and problems with short-term memory—inability to follow directions

Confusion—suddenly becomes uncomfortable in familiar surroundings

Dizzy spells—falling down and blurred vision issues—always in a hurry—rush, rush, rush—still walks three miles three times a week.

Daily headaches—loses track of how many Excedrin he has taken

Agitated mood swings with lack of concentration, communication challenges and difficulty solving problems—frequently yells at family members in public—constantly discusses politics as though he's looking for a verbal fight—he's always right and things must be done his way

Body thermostat is off—75 degrees outside and he has the heat on in the summer

Pushes his way to the front of the line oblivious to others following courteous protocol

Can fall asleep easily throughout the day—sleepless nights

Diabetes—constantly harping that he's allergic to sugar

Always forgetting to zip up his pants

Frequent ear pain affecting his mood—blasts the TV thinking it will keep him awake, but it doesn't; then he's upset again

Continues to drive long distances; climbs ladders and picks fruit. Has no peripheral vision. Family concerned for him and others on the road

Continues to be more unreasonable with each passing day.

John's family has developed several techniques to help deal with him.

1. Always treat the person with respect and listen to his/her side of the story
2. Offer praise for appropriate and safe behavior (e.g., "You really handled that situation well; I'm so glad you decided to ask someone to pick you up.")
3. Allow the person to choose among appropriate and safe choices
4. Be assertive and set necessary limits. Explain your concerns and feelings in a supportive way.

My father-in-law lives in our home. My wife is the one most responsible for his well being on a daily basis. She is much more than a caregiver. Listen to her story—maybe you will hear some of your own family experiences. She writes the following.

"My 94-year-old father lives in our home. Over the past few years, Dad began spending increasingly frequent and more extended periods of time with us. He had lived alone in our family home for eight years following my mother's death. It was our family home for 46 years. With the upkeep and stairs, it became obvious that it was too difficult and dangerous for him to continue to live there alone. For Dad, coming to live in Iowa was "a natural". Although he lived the vast majority of his life in Chicago, he was born in Iowa and spent many summers as a child and young man with cousins and family on the farm. He cherishes many great memories from those long ago days.

I continue to respect and honor my father as the man who raised, taught, and provided for me. I am his daughter as well as his caregiver. I do not like that term, as I merely provide for my father what many adult children who love their parent and have the ability would do. My father is not my patient. My home is not a care facility. It is now home to my husband and me as well as my father and our two dogs. We meet each other's needs as they arise.

That said there are adjustments I have had to make to accommodate my father. I am a registered nurse, but have cut my work hours back drastically. My employer has been very accommodating to my situation. When I do work outside our home, I have a woman who spends a good portion of the day with Dad, mostly in a companionship role. We have a first floor room in our house that easily became a bedroom for Dad. I have acquired many of the physical necessities to aid in Dad's comfort. He uses a walker and is very unsteady without it. I help him get into the shower and give him some assistance bathing. The VA has been wonderful in providing assistance and equipment. There have been times that Dad has required more help from me than others, but thankfully his needs are pretty routine at this point. Recently, I bought Dad a power lift chair, which is great assistance.

Despite Dad's advanced age, his mind is still quite sharp. His body, however, has begun to betray him. He most recently endured stomach cancer, which was incidentally found very early and completely removed—an otherwise deadly diagnosis. He's had a few TIA's in the past year, but those have passed for now. He's had diabetes for years that is controlled by medicine. He's had a number of falls, one fairly nasty, but has recovered well each time.

I do not find that caring for my father is the terribly burdensome role people suggest—mostly because Dad's health is pretty stable. I also have a supportive husband. I am no saint and have had to manage a number of emotions to come to this point. I grew up in a family that was taught the Lord comes first. Family comes next. Growing up, both of my grandmothers lived in our home for periods of time so it was not a foreign concept to have Dad live with us. We have always been a close family. I have four younger siblings who are supportive and helpful. Unfortunately, they all live more than 300 miles away. Dad came to live with me because my time is the most flexible.

I have come to know my dad so much better as the months and years have passed with him in our home. He shares stories of his youth and defining times of his life including his many World War II experiences. My own adult children get to spend more time with Grandpa. He even counsels them in their careers and is able to translate his own work experience to their computer age worlds. My daughter often stays with "Pop" for an evening when my husband and I have an outing.

For many years I lived far from home, so for me this is a time to give to my father and my family in a real and valuable way. I take my dad to church, to appointments, and he accompanies me as we run errands. He's even been in my daughter's backyard hot tub. I help Dad with his finances and his mail and many daily activities. I surely do not suggest this is all easy, nor is this arrangement right for everyone. But it is manageable and with the help of the Lord we see our way through each day and trust in His care as the future unfolds."

Do you see yourself in her words? Are you a "caregiver", a son, a daughter, a health care worker, a nurse, a doctor, pharmacist or preacher? Aren't we all part of the picture? Don't we all hope and pray that if we are so blessed to reach age 90, that we have someone who "cares" for us and "gives" of his or herself to make our lives meaningful?

Chapter 10

What's Wrong with My Body Doc?

As we age our bodies change in important ways that make medical care more difficult. Obviously at age 90 these bodily changes will be very evident. Aging makes blood vessels stiff and noncompliant. The walls of the blood vessels thicken and scar. The heart muscle often thickens and scars as it tries to pump blood into these "old arteries". As a cardiologist I see this as high blood pressure and heart failure. Thus it is normal for blood pressure to increase with age, especially the top number, which we call systolic blood pressure. Studies have shown us that what is normal at age 30 may be too low at age 90, and if we insist erroneously that we must achieve these umbers, we can cause great harm. An example would be dizziness or black out spells. Likewise, failure of the heart looks different at age 90. Often our traditional markers and tests look normal and more sophisticated testing is needed to clarify the situation. We have learned that mild to moderate obesity in the very elderly is not the risk factor it is in younger folks. I tell patients, "It's better to be fat and fit than skinny and sitting on your fanny." It's true. Keep moving; don't sit around. If you have weighed 200 pounds all your adult life, age 90 is not the time to go on a diet. Instead, eat what you have eaten all these years, but move, move, and move. In fact, the alarm goes off when patients tell me they can't maintain their normal weight and just aren't hungry anymore. That is a real red flag!

As a cardiologist, I do see heart rhythm problems increase as people age, especially one that goes by the ominous name of atrial fibrillation. This makes the heart rhythm irregular and the heart beat fast. It can cause all sorts of distress. How we treat it depends on how disabling it is to the person. Sometimes we need to shock the heart back into rhythm or consider long term use of blood thinners referred to as anticoagulants.

The use of anticoagulants has inherent risk regardless of age, but in the very elderly with the risk of falls it can be a treatment nightmare. Here the concept of risk-benefit and do no harm becomes real and paramount. There is no book I can refer to—it is a judgment in consultation with the patient and family where treatment guidelines often take a back seat to common sense.

I often have to ask myself, "Should I treat all these medical issues with a whole handful of medications, complicated instructions, and unrealistic expectations? Or should I let some of the issues just slide? What is it I'm trying to do anyway? How am I trying best to help this individual? Will this patient just get confused and quit all the medications? Does it really matter if his cholesterol is too high? It's hard enough for the person just to remember to take medications, let alone know all the names and side effects." That's my job.

By the way, do you really know how your car works? Isn't it enough to remember to fill the tank with gas, wear your seat belt, turn on the lights and get the oil changed now and then?

My job is to simplify patients' medications, try to help improve the quality of their lives, and keep it all in the context of patient and family's attitudes and values, not mine. Should they take vitamins? Maybe. But not too much. Keep it simple. Perhaps just one "over 50" multivitamin will do just fine.

Should Mr. Jones carry nitroglycerin for the possibility he might have chest pain? Maybe. But will it lower his blood pressure too much? After all, he uses a walker and his eyesight is poor and he can't keep his medications straight to begin with and by the way, he hates taking medicines.

Should Mary have a pacemaker? Her heart rate is very slow. It might help. Is she active? Does she just sit around? What does she think? Can she figure out how to call in for pacemaker follow-up? Does she live in town? Can her son drive her to her appointments? Will it improve the quality of her life?

How about Al? He had a heart attack 15 years ago. He was left with considerable heart damage. He is getting by. According to today's criteria he would qualify for a fancy pacemaker including a device called a defibrillator. Just look at the criteria, it says it right there in black and white bold type. But really, common sense says no way. Is he living on borrowed time? Obviously. But aren't we all?

In my practice of cardiology these are the types of daily issues that involve the care of the very elderly. They used to be the kinds of problems I would address once a week, but now it is two to three times per day. It is not just medicine; it is our society as a whole. We continue to glorify youth and vigor, but we as a nation are getting old.

Chapter 11

Doctor, Don't Abandon Me

I would like to get a bit more personal now. After all, I am a doctor with my own story and biased thinking, based partly on experience, frustration, and lessons learned.

It is not just cliché to say, "I have learned from my patients." I really have! What is medically appropriate at age 60 often is not at appropriate at age 90. With so many expensive tests, procedures, and gadgets it is a daily struggle. Am I being too aggressive? Am I denying care? So called "Appropriate Use Criteria" prevent fraudulent abuse of truly wasteful or unnecessary testing, but do not address age and common sense. Any decision-making should include family members if they are available. However, this should not be done on the sly or in an attempt to exclude the patient's input.

A good example of a common problem is one I referred to in the previous chapter. That is the decision whether to insert a $60,000 device that can shock the heart back into normal rhythm if a lethal heart rhythm should occur out of the blue. Certain criteria must be met before payers will allow insertion of the device. That's the easy part. The hard part is being the patient's advocate, and in a sense, getting inside their brain, and figuring out if this makes sense. What is the quality of their life? Not my definition, but their definition.

Have they given verbal clues? Can they do the prescribed follow-up? Am I silly even to consider this device at age 90? Should I be blind to age? I am conservative by nature in testing and ordering expensive medications. Does this affect me in regard to this patient? Probably. Should I run the case by one of my partners? Sometimes the patient helps me out. "Doc, I don't want no pacemaker in my chest. When it's time to go the good Lord can just take me." Whew, dodged another bullet.

Frailty is another marker of nearing the end of life that is hard to deal with and give appropriate care and counseling. It is usually characterized by increasing fatigue, weight loss, low blood proteins, anemia, frequent falls, and a general withdrawal from the joys of life. It may be a disease process continuing its relentless grind toward a certain end, but often it is a message from the patient. "I have had enough. Please let me alone. I am at peace. I am on my way home to meet my Maker." I realize this more and more as I get older. I don't push patients with pleasantries or more medications. I listen. I try to ask about what is important to them, how do they see things going, should we stop some of their medications, and "will those Hawkeyes finally win a game this weekend?" I always, always give them a return appointment and usually quip, "See you next year, Lord willing; I will be here, so I expect you to be here also."

One of the more challenging daily issues with very elderly patients is the use of the various medications we have at our disposal. Often the doses required are smaller and the chance of drug-drug interaction increases. The desired end points we are trying to achieve will change with age. For instance, what is a desirable blood pressure for someone age 90 versus someone age 40. It is different. At age 90 a blood pressure of 150/80 is great; at age 40 it is too high. At age 90 I'm more concerned about letting blood pressure get too low, then a dizzy spell, a fall, a broken hip, a trip to the hospital, a blood clot, and so it goes. Should I treat high cholesterol at age 90?

Maybe. Maybe not. It depends. Should I treat my patient with a blood thinner to prevent clots in the heart? Certain conditions like atrial fibrillation say we should. But what if Joe lives alone, uses a walker, has falling episodes, and no family around—probably not.

If Martha is a somewhat plump lady of 250 pounds, should I put her on a diet? Probably not. Whatever she has eaten for 90 years seems to have worked so far; why change now?

If Harry comes in and tells me he's smoked a pack of Marlboro's per day for seventy years, should I ask him to quit? Probably not. Will I get a "red frown face" on my assessment from the payers—yes.

The point is that what is good medicine and common sense change as we age. We must concede that these 90 year olds are different than most of us. They have proved it. Our job is just to make sure that silly little things don't side track them. Let them do quirky things. Make sure they wear a seat belt and get a flu shot. Have them bring in their medication list. Have them take a nap, say a prayer, read the paper. Chances are they will come back to see me next year.

Chapter 12

We are All Getting Old—What Does It Mean as a Nation and a Society

We as a nation are getting old. By the year 2030 one in five of us will be 65 years or older. The number of persons living past age 85 will quadruple. The average life expectancy in the United States is now 79 years. Women live longer than men on the average. Females' life expectancy is now 81 years—the mean about 76 years.

It has been estimated that the current lifetime cost of health care in this country exceeds $300,000 per person. Half of this healthcare bill occurs after age 65 and if one lives to be 85, one third of their total health care costs will be used to extend their lives.

In the state of Iowa where I reside, we are really old. Only North Dakota has a higher percentage of its population older than 65. As a physician, this is real life stuff. My primary responsibility is to my patients, regardless of age, but I realize that consequences of the decisions I make for society as a whole. When someone is 90 and they come to see me, it really is about quality of life, not what I think, but what they think. A recent Institute of Medicine study estimated that 70% of patients never talked to their doctor about end of life care and more than 40% had no Advance Directives. The same study showed that when directly queried about life-sustaining therapy, 80% would reject it. The problem is that we as physicians are not very good at asking patients directly about their desires in this area. I know it makes me squeamish. I don't want to stop offering care too soon. Patients do want to help make these decisions. Families want to make these decisions. Four in five elderly patients want to die at home with their family, but sadly, almost one-third die in the ICU. That's the disconnect. It costs a lot in terms of suffering, family stress, and the price tag to society is immense.

In 2010 healthcare spending for the elderly was $18,424 per year per person. At that time they comprised about 13% of the population but consumed 34% of the healthcare dollars. "Cost" is a tricky thing. It's not just dollars spent; it's lives changed. It's playing bridge with friends, having time with grandkids, going to the store, watching old reruns. That's what we hope we all have when we get old.

The reality is that most don't. Male suicide is increasing in frequency in those over age 85. The causes are obvious, yet unsettling and uncomfortable for us to discuss as a society. Social isolation, disability, loss of autonomy, loss of purpose, all are accentuated and most of these issues just won't go away.

As a doctor it's my job to practice what I preach. My job and society's responsibility are to sit down and hash some of these issues out. It takes time. It's not sexy. It can't be delegated, but it must be done. We all hope to grow old gracefully and with dignity. We each have a responsibility to do this in our own families. Yes, it's the right thing to do.

Epilogue

It is now one year later and I'm still working full time and Grandpa is living with us full time. My wife is his full time nurse, confidant, cook, bible study leader, and assists with his finances. He seems happy, content and still loves life. His four other adult children who do not live in the area Skype with him at least once a week. Our daughter comes over several times a week to brighten his day. He still reads the paper, does some crossword puzzles and watches old reruns of The Lawrence Welk Show. His mind is sharp. He can't hear very well but I'm not sure that's important. He sleeps soundly at night and takes two long naps each day. He likes to tease our two little dogs. We don't wonder any longer why Sophie, one of our Shih Tzu's is gaining weight as we catch Grandpa feeding her potato chips from the table.

Several weeks ago an incident occurred that we feared might end Grandpa's placid existence in our home. He was walking with his walker to go to his room. As he walked by the stairs leading to the lower level he got momentary weakness in his knees. You guessed it—down the stairs he went. Both my wife and I were within feet of him, but couldn't help. He slid down 16 stairs, and then did a complete tumble, striking his head, shoulder, and thigh. We rushed after him. He was alive. He was stunned and groggy. We had him just rest there for what seemed an eternity. Big welts were already forming. We called our daughter and her boyfriend to help get him up all the stairs.

The next week was touch and go. A huge hematoma on his head drained down and covered half his face in various colors. The shoulder was obviously injured—he could not raise his arm much. For the next week my wife got very little sleep. She checked on him all night long, every night. But ever so gradually he improved. The swelling began to subside, the purple bruising turned yellow and faded. He began using his arm more and getting strength back. He could get out of bed on his own, and he continued to rally. Wouldn't you know it; a few weeks later he took a bike ride! What a man! God is good indeed. That is my story. I hope you enjoyed the journey.

Bibliography

USA Today for The Des Moines Register. Sunday, June 29, 2014. Julie Appleby, Kaiser Health News.

The Des Moines Register, Sunday, February 22, 2015, Rana Moustafa, IowaWatch.org.

NEJM 372; February 12, 2015. Pizzo and Walker, "Should we practice what we profess?"

JAMA 2013; 310(18) 1947-1964, Hamilton Moses et.al.

Health Services Research. June 2004; 39(3): 627-642.

CMS.gov NHE, 2013.

CPSIA information can be obtained at www.ICGtesting.com
Printed in the USA
LVOW08s0820300516

490437LV00002B/162/P